STEPS TO RECOVERY FROM SUBSTANCE USE

Reclaiming Your Life

Michel Montalvo

Table of Contents

Steps to Recovery from Substance Use

Overview

Addiction is a complex disease that significantly impacts individuals and their loved ones. It can manifest through substance use or compulsive behaviors that lead to detrimental consequences.

Recovery is a multifaceted journey toward health and wellness that often requires support, dedication, and a willingness to change.

Purpose of the Guide

This book serves as a structured guide for individuals seeking to reclaim their lives after substance use. The three-month plan is designed to help readers develop healthy habits, find support, and cultivate resilience.

Setting the Tone

This guide emphasizes hope, growth, and transformation. Each chapter provides practical strategies, emotional support, and a roadmap to achieving a fulfilling life beyond addiction.

Your Journey Begins

As you embark on this transformative journey, remember that you are not alone. Many have walked this path and emerged stronger. Let's begin the journey together!

Month 1:
Foundation of Recovery

The Science of Addiction

Addiction is defined as a chronic, relapsing disorder characterized by compulsive drug seeking, continued use despite harmful consequences, and long-lasting changes in the brain. The brain's reward system becomes altered, leading to changes in mood, behavior, and cognitive function.

Neurobiology of Addiction

Substances can increase the release of dopamine, creating feelings of pleasure. Over time, the brain adapts, requiring more of the substance to achieve the same effect. This cycle perpetuates dependency and hinders the ability to experience joy without the substance.

Personal Stories of Recovery

Stories of individuals who have successfully navigated addiction can be powerful motivators. For example, Sarah struggled with opioid dependency for years but found strength in a supportive community, illustrating that recovery is possible with the right resources.

Broader Impacts of Addiction

Addiction affects not only the individual but also family members, friends, and communities. Understanding these impacts can deepen your resolve to seek recovery, as it not only changes your life but can also mend relationships and improve the lives of those around you.

The Importance of Understanding Addiction

Recognizing that addiction is a disease rather than a personal failure is crucial. This understanding can help dismantle stigma and encourage compassion for oneself and others on the recovery journey.

Initial Steps to Recovery

Acknowledgment of the Problem

The first step in recovery is acknowledging that a problem exists. This admission can be difficult, but it's essential for initiating change. Reflect on your behaviors and their consequences to fully grasp the need for recovery.

Setting Personal Goals

Once you've acknowledged your situation, establishing clear, achievable goals is the next step. Identify what recovery looks like for you, whether it's abstaining from substances, improving health, or rebuilding relationships.

SMART Goals Explained

Utilize the SMART criteria to create effective goals:
- Specific: Clearly define your objectives.
- Measurable: Identify how you will track progress.
- Achievable: Ensure your goals are realistic given your current circumstances.
- Relevant: Align your goals with your values and long-term aspirations.
- Time-bound: Set deadlines for your goals to maintain accountability.

Example of a SMART Goal

Instead of saying, "I want to quit drinking," articulate a SMART goal: "I will attend three AA meetings each week for the next month to support my sobriety."

Commitment to Your Goals

Write down your goals and revisit them regularly. This commitment serves as a constant reminder of your intentions and helps reinforce your motivation.

Daily Routines
Establishing Morning Rituals

Creating a structured morning routine can significantly impact your mindset for the day. Consider waking up at the same time each day to promote consistency.

Meditation as a Morning Practice

Begin each day with 10 minutes of mindfulness meditation. Focus on your breath and allow thoughts to come and go without judgment. This practice can enhance self-awareness and reduce anxiety.

Journaling for Clarity

Follow meditation with 15 minutes of journaling. Write down three things you are grateful for and set positive intentions for the day ahead. Gratitude can shift your focus from negativity to positivity.

Nutrition and Meal Planning

Nutrition is vital during recovery. Create a meal plan emphasizing whole foods—fruits, vegetables, lean proteins, and whole grains. These foods can improve mood and overall health.

Sample Meal Plan

- Breakfast: Overnight oats with berries and nuts.
- Lunch: Quinoa salad with grilled chicken and mixed vegetables.
- Dinner: Baked fish with steamed broccoli and sweet potatoes.
- Snacks: Fresh fruit, yogurt, or nuts.

Support Systems
The Importance of Support Groups

Connecting with others who understand your struggles is crucial. Support groups like Alcoholics Anonymous (AA) offer a safe space to share experiences and learn from one another.

Therapy Options

In addition to support groups, consider seeking therapy. A licensed professional can provide valuable insights and tools to navigate your recovery journey.

Building a Sober Network

Surround yourself with people who support your recovery efforts. This network can include friends, family, or new acquaintances met through support groups.

Effective Communication

Be open and honest with those you trust about your journey. Sharing your feelings and experiences can create deeper connections and accountability.

Finding an Accountability Partner

Consider finding someone to share your recovery goals with—an accountability partner who can encourage you and help you stay on track.

Mindfulness and Coping Strategies

Practicing Mindfulness

Mindfulness helps manage stress and cravings. Engage in mindfulness meditation regularly to cultivate awareness of the present moment.

Breathing Exercises for Calmness

Deep breathing techniques can help alleviate anxiety. Inhale deeply for four counts, hold for four counts, and exhale slowly for six counts. Repeat this several times to feel grounded.

Grounding Techniques

Use grounding exercises to stay present during cravings. Try the "5-4-3-2-1" technique: Identify 5 things you can see, 4 things you can touch, 3 things you can hear, 2 things you can smell, and 1 thing you can taste.

Reflective Journaling

Set aside time each evening for reflective journaling. Write about your feelings, challenges faced, and successes of the day to reinforce positive experiences.

Utilizing Mindfulness Apps

Explore mindfulness apps such as Insight Timer or Simple Habit for guided meditation sessions that can assist in establishing a consistent practice.

Month 2: Building Strength and Resilience

Cognitive-Behavioral Strategies

Cognitive-behavioral therapy (CBT) can help you identify and change negative thought patterns that contribute to substance use. Understanding these thoughts is essential for effective coping.

Identifying Triggers

Keep a journal to document situations, emotions, and thoughts that trigger cravings. Awareness of triggers is the first step toward managing them effectively.

Developing Healthy Coping Strategies

Create a list of alternative activities to engage in when cravings hit. This could include going for a walk, reading, or practicing a hobby that brings you joy.

Incorporating Positive Affirmations

Use positive affirmations to bolster your self-esteem and reinforce your commitment to recovery. Repeat phrases like "I am strong," or "I can overcome challenges."

Seeking Professional Guidance

Consider working with a therapist trained in CBT to help you develop and implement these strategies effectively.

Daily Routines
Rediscovering Hobbies

Engaging in hobbies can provide healthy distractions and a sense of accomplishment. Explore activities that you once enjoyed or try something new.

Suggestions for Hobbies

- Painting or drawing
- Playing a musical instrument
- Writing or journaling
- Cooking or baking

Increasing Exercise Intensity

As you become more comfortable with physical activity, increase the intensity of your workouts. Experiment with new forms of exercise, such as dance classes or group sports.

Sample Weekly Exercise Plan

- Monday: 30 minutes of yoga
- Tuesday: 20 minutes of brisk walking
- Wednesday: Dance class
- Thursday: Bodyweight strength training
- Friday: Outdoor activity (hiking or biking)

Listening to Your Body's Needs

Pay attention to how your body feels during and after exercise. Rest and recover when needed, and celebrate small victories in your fitness journey.

Alternative Therapies

Exploring Yoga

Yoga is a holistic practice that can enhance both physical and mental well-being. Look for beginner classes in your community or online platforms.

Benefits of Yoga in Recovery

- Increases flexibility and strength
- Reduces stress and anxiety
- Promotes mindfulness and self-awareness

Beginner Yoga Poses

- Child's Pose: A restful pose that encourages relaxation and deep breathing.
- Downward Dog: A foundational pose that strengthens and stretches the body.
- Corpse Pose: A restorative pose that promotes deep relaxation and grounding.

Considering Acupuncture

Acupuncture has been shown to help reduce cravings and anxiety in individuals recovering from substance use. Look for licensed practitioners in your area.

Researching Other Alternative Therapies

Explore additional alternative therapies such as aromatherapy, massage therapy, or art therapy to find what resonates with you.

Nutrition and Wellness

Focus on Balanced Meals

A nutritious diet supports recovery by promoting physical and mental health. Prioritize whole, unprocessed foods and limit sugar and caffeine.

Sample Recipes for Recovery

- Breakfast: Smoothie with spinach, banana, and almond milk.
- Lunch: Lentil soup with a side salad.
- Dinner: Stir-fried vegetables with tofu and brown rice.

Importance of Hydration

Staying hydrated is crucial for overall health. Aim for at least 8 glasses of water a day, and consider herbal teas as a comforting alternative.

Discussing Supplements with Healthcare Providers

Consult a healthcare provider about supplements that may support your recovery. Options like Omega-3 fatty acids and B vitamins can be beneficial.

Creating a Weekly Meal Plan

Develop a meal plan that incorporates a variety of nutrient-dense foods. Preparing meals in advance can help you stay on track and reduce stress around mealtime.

Reflective Practices
Gratitude Journaling

Establish a gratitude journaling practice by noting three things you are thankful for each day. This simple practice can enhance your mood and perspective.

Regular Check-Ins with Support Networks

Schedule regular therapy sessions or support group meetings to discuss your progress and any challenges you encounter.

Engaging in Self-Reflection

Spend time each week reflecting on what you've learned about yourself during your recovery. This practice can foster self-awareness and growth.

Adapting Coping Strategies

Be open to adjusting your coping strategies as you learn what works best for you. Recovery is a dynamic process that requires flexibility.

Celebrating Your Achievements

Recognize and celebrate even the smallest victories in your recovery journey. Acknowledging progress is vital for maintaining motivation.

Month 3: Reinforcing Your New Life

Creating a Long-Term Plan

Setting Future Goals

Consider your long-term vision for life after recovery. Write down personal and professional goals that inspire you, envisioning where you want to be in six months, a year, and beyond.

Creating a Vision Board

A vision board can help you visualize your goals. Use images, quotes, and items that represent your aspirations, placing it somewhere you can see daily to maintain motivation.

Developing a Relapse Prevention Plan

Create a personalized relapse prevention plan that identifies triggers and outlines strategies for managing them effectively. This plan should be a living document that you review regularly.

Listing Emergency Contacts

Compile a list of emergency contacts, including trusted friends, family, and support group members. Keep this list handy for times when you need support or encouragement.

Building Resilience through Reflection

Reflect on challenges you've faced during recovery and how you've overcome them. This exercise builds confidence in your ability to navigate future obstacles.

Daily Routines
Consistency in Routines

Establishing consistent daily routines can promote stability. Set specific times for waking up, meals, exercise, and self-care to create a predictable structure.

Sample Daily Schedule

- 7:00 AM: Wake up and meditate
- 7:30 AM: Eat a healthy breakfast
- 8:00 AM: Engage in morning exercise
- 9:00 AM: Focus on work or personal projects
- 12:00 PM: Have lunch and take a short walk
- 1:00 PM: Continue afternoon activities
- 5:00 PM: Prepare and enjoy dinner
- 7:00 PM: Evening self-care routine (reading, journaling)

Designating Self-Care Days

Incorporate regular self-care days into your routine. Dedicate time to activities that rejuvenate you, such as visiting a spa, going for a hike, or simply relaxing at home.

Prioritizing Sleep for Recovery

Aim for 7-9 hours of quality sleep each night. Establish a calming bedtime routine to improve sleep quality and support your recovery process.

Flexibility in Your Routines

Be adaptable with your routines. Life can be unpredictable, and it's essential to adjust while remaining committed to your recovery.

Community Engagement

The Value of Volunteering

Volunteering can provide a sense of purpose and fulfillment. Research local organizations that resonate with your values and interests.

Benefits of Volunteering

- Enhances social connections and community involvement

- Provides a sense of accomplishment and fulfillment

- It helps develop new skills and perspectives

Participating in Sober Activities

Seek out local sober events and gatherings, such as movie nights, game nights, or community clean-ups. Engaging in sober activities can help build a supportive network.

Joining Clubs or Classes

Consider joining clubs or taking classes that align with your interests. Whether it's a book club, art class, or sports league, these activities can foster new friendships.

Cultivating Relationships with Supportive Individuals

Focus on building friendships with those who support your recovery journey. Quality relationships can have a profound impact on your well-being.

Continued Learning and Growth

Expanding Your Knowledge

Educate yourself about addiction and recovery through books, articles, and reputable online resources. Knowledge empowers you to make informed decisions.

Recommended Reading List

- "The Recovery Book" by Al Mooney, M.D.: A comprehensive guide to strategies for recovery.
- "Addiction Recovery Management" by John F. Kelly: Insights into the ongoing process of managing recovery.

Attending Workshops
and Retreats

Look for workshops or retreats focused on personal growth and recovery. These experiences can provide valuable tools and insights.

Exploring Online Courses

Consider enrolling in online courses that focus on mindfulness, emotional intelligence, or stress management. These resources can deepen your understanding and enhance your coping skills.

Investing in Personal Development

Set aside time for personal development. Pursue new interests or skills that excite you, contributing to your overall growth and fulfillment.

Celebrating Progress

Recognizing Milestones in Recovery

Celebrate your achievements, big and small. Recognizing milestones fosters a sense of accomplishment and reinforces your commitment to recovery.

Planning a Celebration for Your Sobriety

Organize a celebration to honor your sobriety journey. Whether it's a gathering with friends or a quiet day reflecting on your progress, make it meaningful.

Reflecting on Your Recovery Journey

Take time to reflect on your journey. Write about your experiences, growth, and what you've learned along the way.

Setting New Goals
for the Future

As you celebrate your accomplishments, set new goals that inspire you. Continuously strive for personal growth and embrace new opportunities.

Embracing a Bright Future

Look forward with optimism and embrace the possibilities ahead. Recovery is a lifelong journey, and every day offers new opportunities for growth and renewal.

The Unique Journey
of Recovery

Your journey through recovery is unique and ongoing. Celebrate the progress you've made and stay committed to your path of self-discovery and healing.

The Holistic Nature
of Recovery

Remember that recovery isn't solely about abstaining from substances; it's about rebuilding your life in a way that fulfills you. Continue to seek support and embrace new experiences.

Resources for Ongoing Support

There are numerous resources available for support. Whether through therapy, support groups, or online communities, don't hesitate to reach out when you need assistance.

Gratitude for Your Journey

Thank you for taking the time to embark on this journey of healing and transformation. You possess the strength to reclaim your life and create a brighter future.

References

- Volkow, N. D., Koob, G. F., & McLellan, A. T. (2016). Neurobiology of addiction: A disease of adaptation. American Journal of Psychiatry, 173(3), 219-233.
- Mooney, A., Mooney, J., & Kahn, M. (2011). The Recovery Book: Answers to All Your Questions About Addiction and Alcoholism and Finding Health and Happiness in Sobriety. Da Capo Press.
- Kelly, J. F., & White, W. L. (2012). Addiction Recovery Management: Theory, Research, and Practice. The Guilford Press.
- Substance Abuse and Mental Health Services Administration (SAMHSA). (2021). Treatment Improvement Protocol (TIP) Series.
- American Psychiatric Association. (2013). Diagnostic and Statistical Manual of Mental Disorders (5th ed.). Arlington, VA: American Psychiatric Publishing.
- Miller, W. R., & Rollnick, S. (2013). Motivational Interviewing: Helping People Change (3rd ed.). Guilford Press.
- Brown, S. A., & Ashcraft, R. (2006). The effects of a structured recovery program on abstinence and quality of life in individuals with alcohol use disorders. Journal of Substance Abuse Treatment, 31(2), 141-149.
- Dackis, M. N., & O'Brien, C. P. (2005). Neurobiology of addiction: A disease of the brain. Journal of Substance Abuse Treatment, 29(1), 41-52.
- Gorski, T. T. (2000). The Relapse Prevention Workbook. The Gorski-CENAPS Model.
- Greenfield, S. F., & Grella, C. E. (2009). Alcohol and drug use disorders. Psychiatric Clinics of North America, 32(3), 433-449.

9 798344 151557